Armour Plated Shoulders

Armour Plated Shoulders

A Training & Maintanance Shoulder Program Specifically Designed for Law Enforcement, Security & First Responders

HARD CORPS™ ATHLETICS Inc.
Program design and development:

Ahmad Soltani

Model: Mark Longshore

ISBN: 1979110751
ISBN 13: 9781979110754

Table of Content

"Ouch, My Shoulder Hurts!"

The shoulder and all its problems

How often do you hear, " I can't lift my arm, my shoulder hurts." Or," I can't get a good nights rest because of this shoulder." The risk of shoulder injury in our culture is relatively high. Of course, the more regular activity a person does, the higher the risk for injury to the shoulder. Almost all first responders and security corps suffer a shoulder cuff injury at some point in their career. The rotator cuff – four small muscles that stabilize the shoulder and help with the rotation of the arm – gets pulled, stretched, and generally bashed about by regular activity. Over time, degeneration of the cuff can limit your shoulders range of movement and leave you with chronic shoulder pain.

The problem has many folds. The shoulder is a complicated joint that can be easily damaged if misused or overused. Without getting into the detailed mechanics of it, we will simply state that without some basic movement training, handling relatively heavy loads (15% of your body weight or higher) in any manner with one or two hands dramatically increases your risk for shoulder injuries. This does not mean that if you lift an equipment bag and throw it in your car you will injure your rotator cuff, but you increase the chance of injury overall – say going to the grocery store afterwards and loading grocery bags in your car.

The good news is that research has improved our understanding of shoulder bio-mechanics and provided the knowledge to dramatically reduce the risk of injury. And if injured, to rehabilitate the damage with exercise and specific movement patterns. Take for example a Lifting a piece of equipment off the ground. Even if the weight is light, not setting your shoulders before you lift, can significantly increase the risk of impingement and inevitable injury. Moreover, it is typical to hear emergency workers, first responders and law enforcement officers complain about painful shoulders.

The good news is that most of these injuries can be prevented. The better news is that it does not take more than a short sessions a week, given the correct exercises and time, to truly amour plate your shoulders and reduce your risk of injury. A purpose driven exercise program is the name of the game. The exercise that specifically targets and benefits the shoulder in general and the rotator cuff in particular are finite and simple to learn. Once you have learned the movements that address you specific needs and put those few movements into a personalized program, all you need is about 10 - 15 minutes a day and you can ARMOUR PLATE your shoulders. Just about everyone suffers from shoulder problems. In this book, I have brought together 7 specific exercises in a pre arranged order to "Armor Plate" your shoulders. With over 25 years of experience in physical training, I have spent a lot of time coming up with solutions for my clients. Given that there is no simple solution to this very complex problem, using these exercises in a weekly program can substantially improve your shoulder strength, stability and mobility. And, because of the added mobility you will reduce the risk of injury.

Specifically designed for Law Enforcement, Security and First Responders, this program targets the shoulder's vulnerabilities due to extreme work conditions. Addressing these areas protects the shoulder from injury while reducing the risk of injury. This is a simple, 45 minutes a week program that will change & improve the way you do your work.

Anatomy of an Impingement

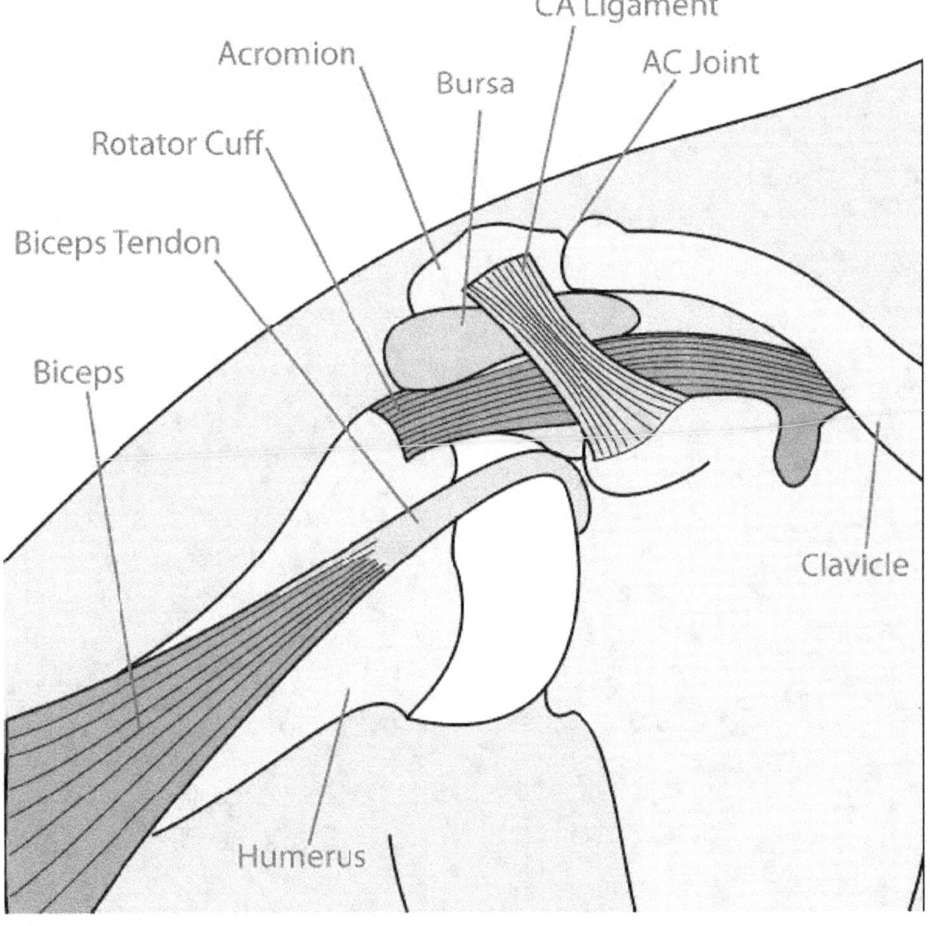

The problem arises when the Rotator Cuff gets pinched between the top of the Humerus and the AC Joint. This is typically referred to as an ***impingement.***

9 Week Training Cycle

WEEK	# of sets/reps	# of workouts
Week 1,2,3	2 sets of 10	2 per week
Week 4,5	2 sets of 14	2 per week
Week 6, 7	2 sets of 18	2 per week
Week 8,9	1 set of 20	2 per week
Maintenance	*2 sets of 12*	*2 - 3 times per week*

GET TO WORK

Setting Your Shoulders

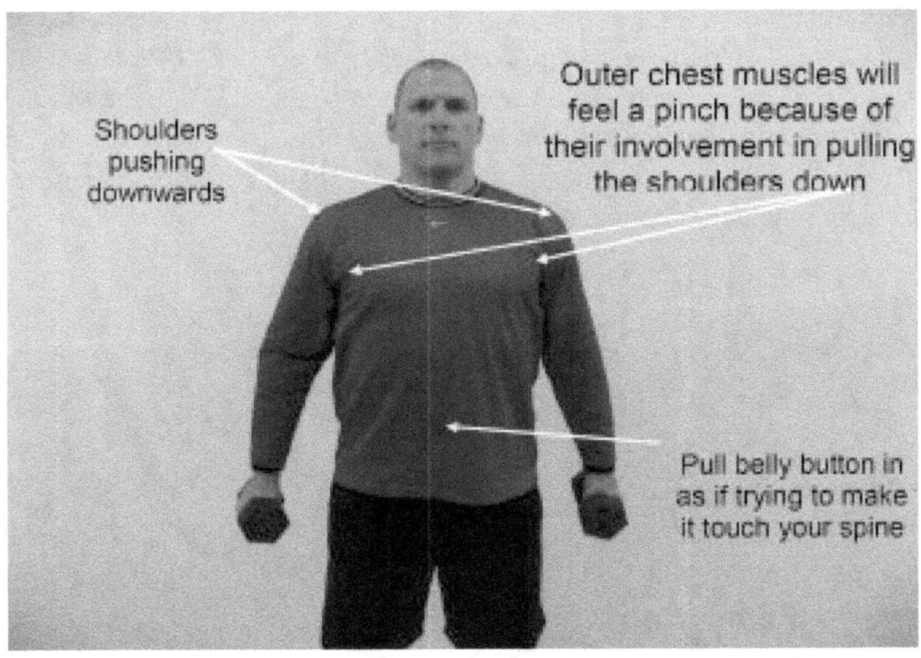

Setting your shoulders is a technique developed by HCA to alleviate shoulder pain due to impingement and to reduce the risk of injury due to improper rotation of the cuffs or other contributing muscles. Follow the next two steps and feel the difference this technique makes when it comes to shoulder movement. Go back to your regular technique to get a clearer idea.

1. *Pull in your belly button by contracting your stomach muscles. You should be able to breath and talk normally as your perform this movement. If correctly done, the result will be a tightening feeling from your hip all the way up and past your rib cage. A useful visualization would be trying to get your belly button to touch your spine.*
2. *Push the shoulders down and hold them there. Note: the shoulders are held in the frontal plane: **Do not** force your shoulders down if they are either sagging to the front or the back. Check your form in the mirror from the side. It will be easy to see if you are not lined up correctly.*

Now your shoulders are set and you are ready to exercise. This technique is applicable to most upper body exercises. As you go through the routine in this program, be sure to set your shoulders before each exercise. As you become familiar with the technique, begin applying it to other exercises involving the upper body.

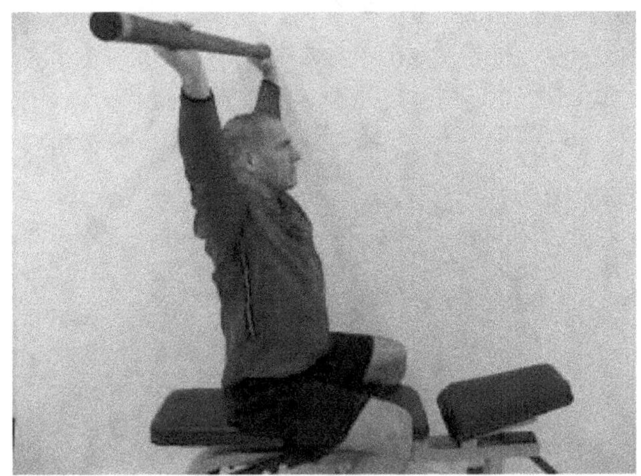

Rear Shoulder Press

- Begin with the weight above your head and slightly behind you.
- Set the shoulders.
- As you begin to lower the weight down, draw you belly button in. This will help you stabilize your torso.
- Stop at the bottom of the movement.
- With your belly button drawn in, press the weight up.
- Repeat with the same pace.

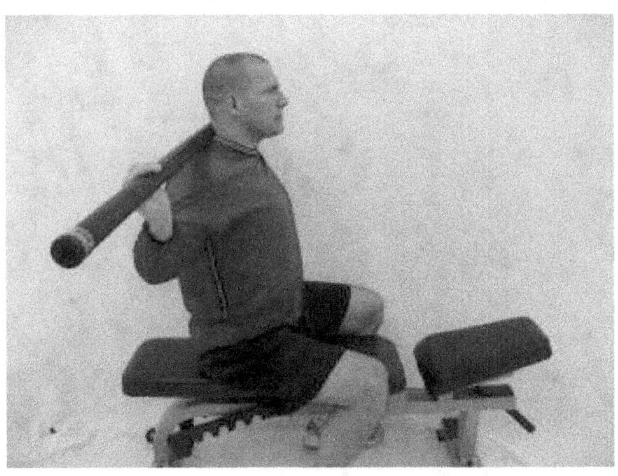

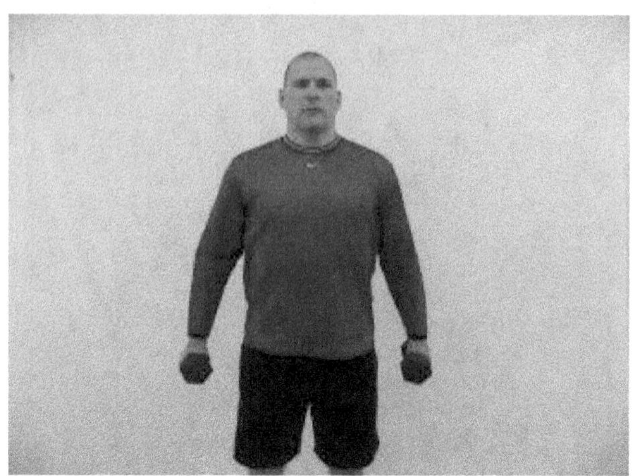

Side Deltoid Raises

- Hold the weights in your hands and set your shoulders.
- With loose grips, begin to raise the weights up to your sides.
- Be sure to keep your hands back—out of your peripheral vision.
- Raise the dumbbells no higher than your shoulders.
- Return and repeat

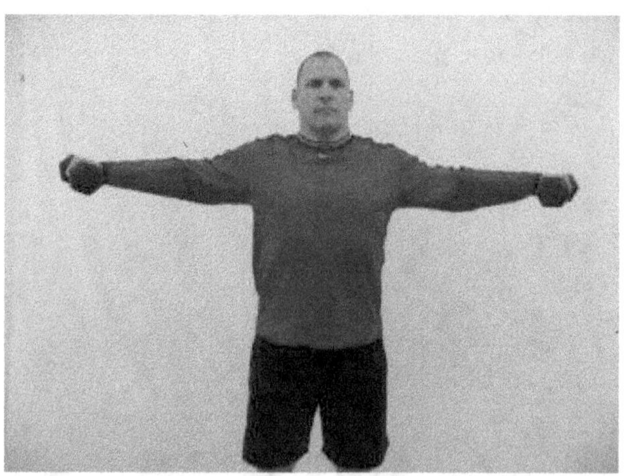

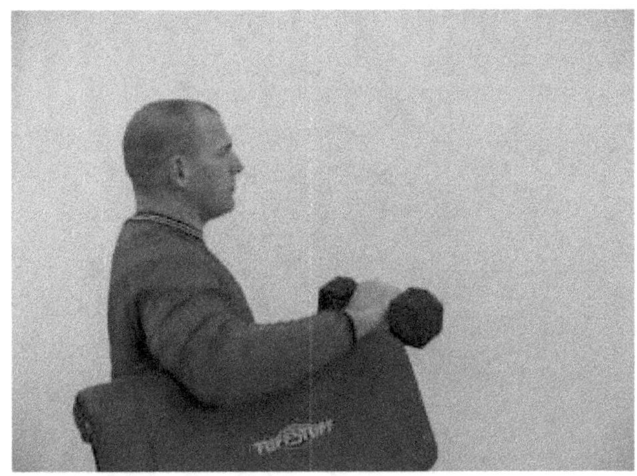

Sitting "L" Flys

- Sit on a bench and rest your elbow on a platform (like below).
- Set your shoulder.
- Begin to lift the dumbbell up toward your shoulder.
- Keep a loose grip.
- Stop when perpendicular, return and repeat.

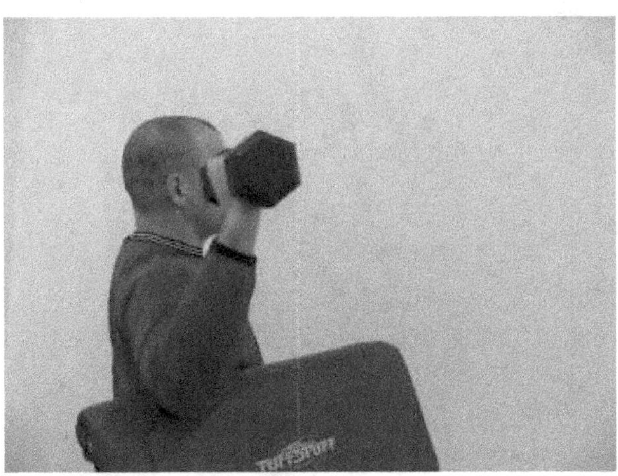

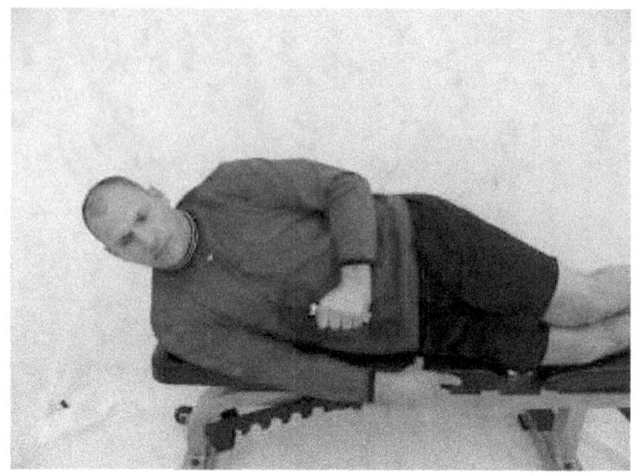

Lying "L" Flys

- Lay on your side, hold the dumbbell gently.
- Set your shoulder.
- With your elbow resting on your side, begin to lift.
- Keep your elbow to your side and continue to lift.
- Stop once perpendicular.
- Return and repeat.

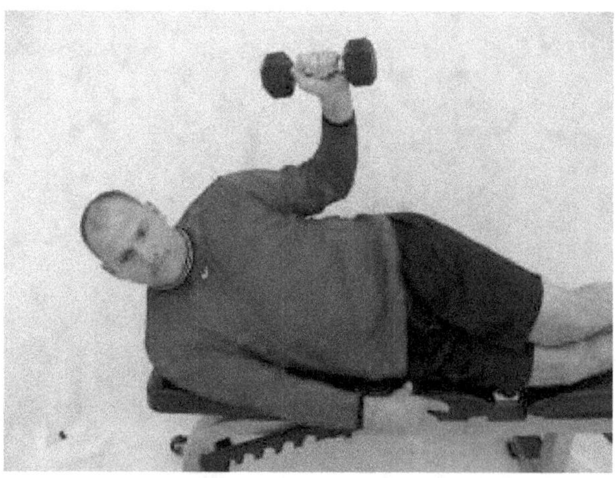

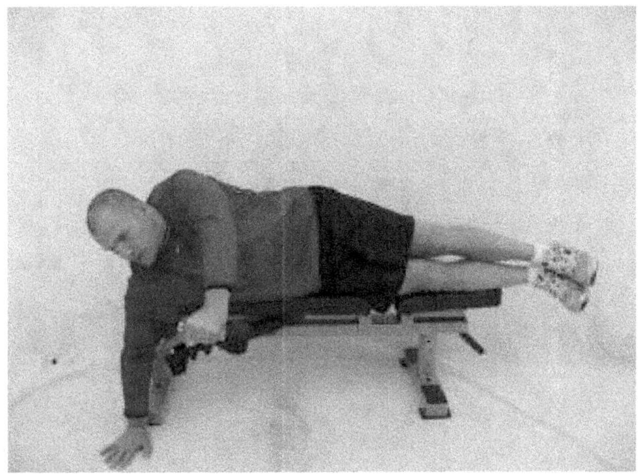

Lying Flys

- Lay on your side on a bench and stabilize yourself with the bottom arm.
- Grip the dumbbell loosely and set your shoulder.
- Gently flex your rear shoulder muscle and begin the lift.
- When you reach the top of the movement stop briefly.
- Return to the bottom and repeat. Maintain the same pace in both directions.

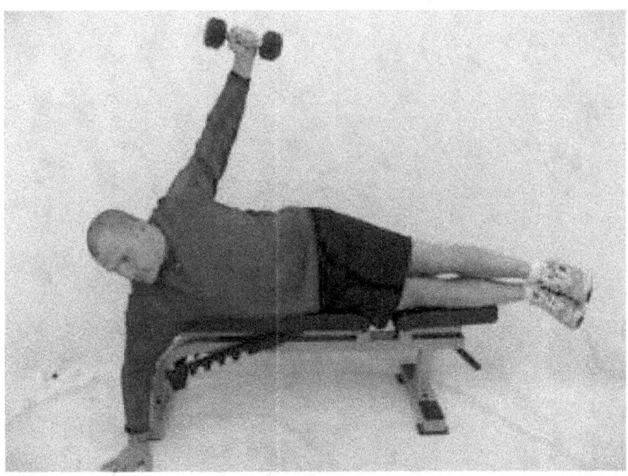

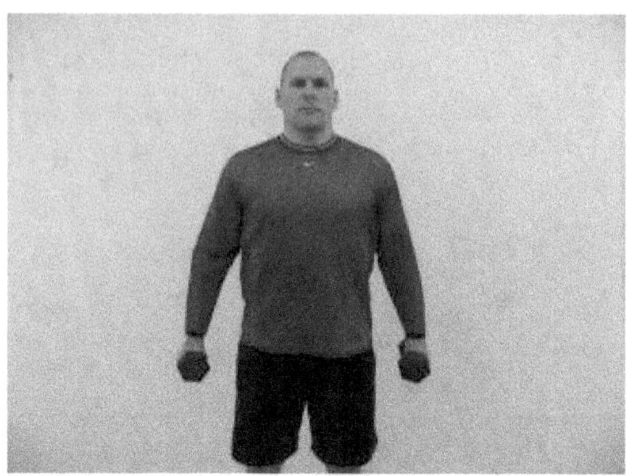

Quarter Eagles

- Hold the weights in your hands and set your shoulders.
- With loose grips, begin to raise the weights forward as you rotate your wrists out (palms up).
- You should feel the force in the arm/torso attachment.
- Stop the rotation when the bottom of the dumbbells are facing out—and no higher than your shoulder level.
- As you return to your original position, rise and twist the opposite direction. Reverse the movement and repeat.
- Maintain the same speed in both directions.

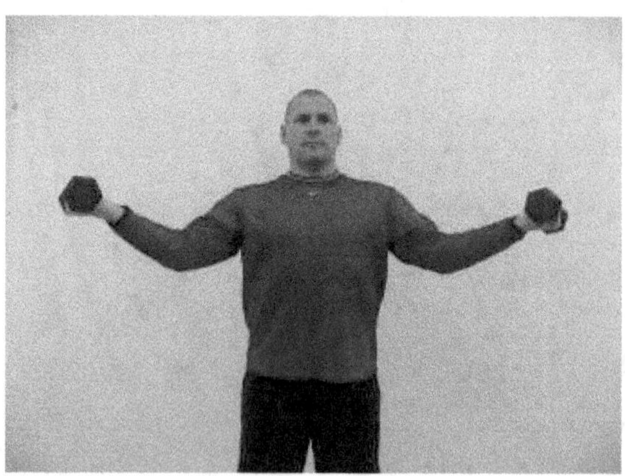

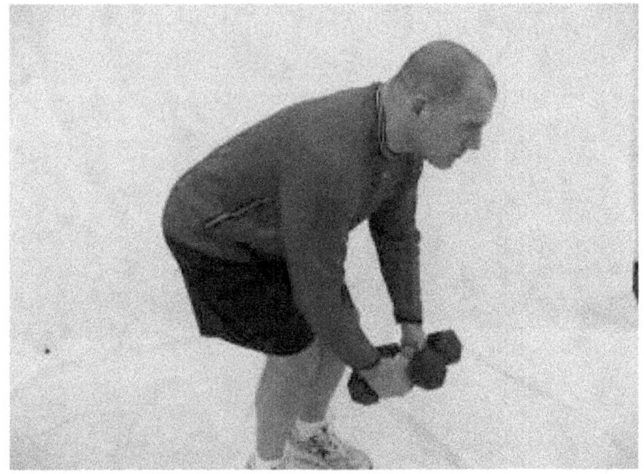

Rear Deltoid Raises

- Stand with the dumbbells lightly in your hand and lean slightly forward. Be sure not to hunch over, this will put too much pressure on your lower back.
- Set your shoulders.
- Begin to lift the dumbbells up by trying to bring your shoulder blades together.
- Raise the dumbbells to your sides. Keep them out of your peripheral vision.
- Hold for a split second, return and repeat.

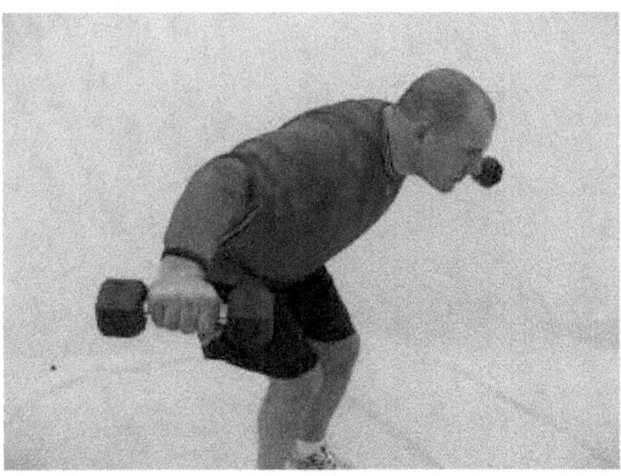

CONDENSED WORKOUT

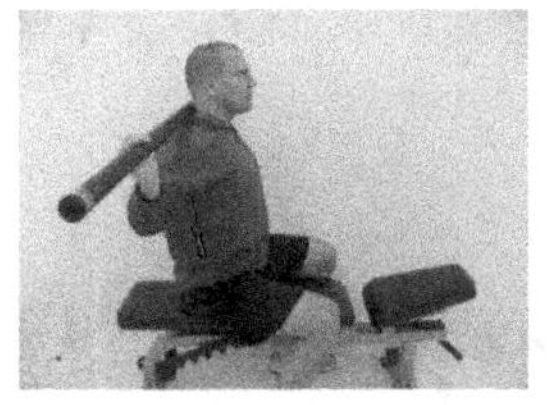 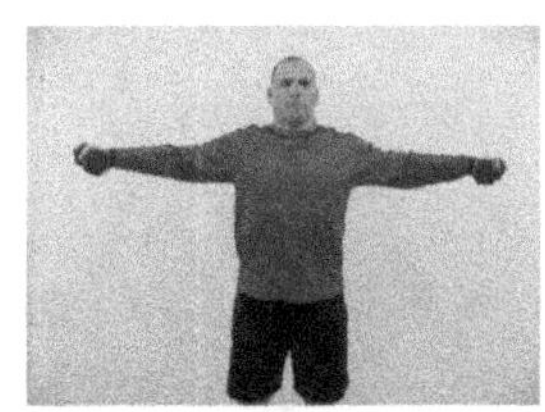

Rear Shoulder Press
2 X 12

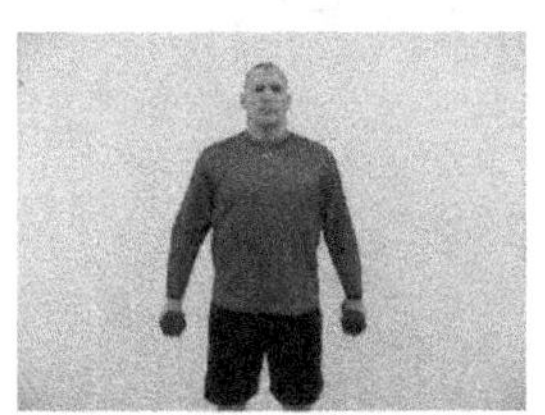 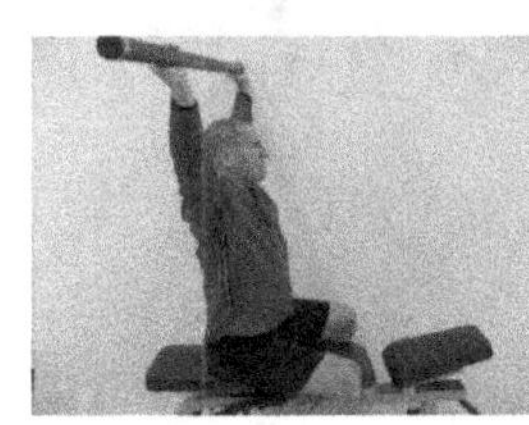

Side Delt Lifts
2 X 12

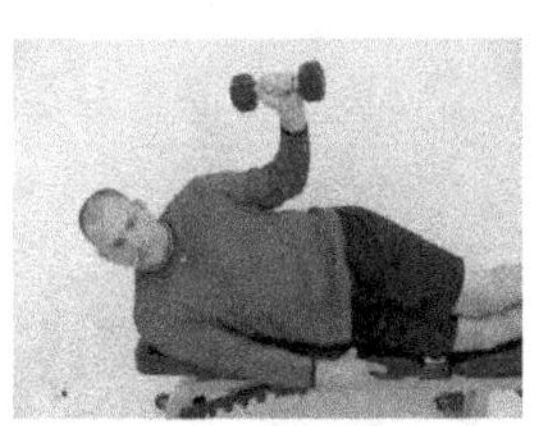 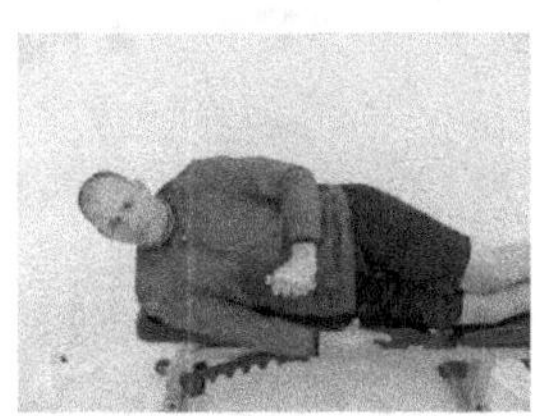

Lying "L" Flys
2 X 12

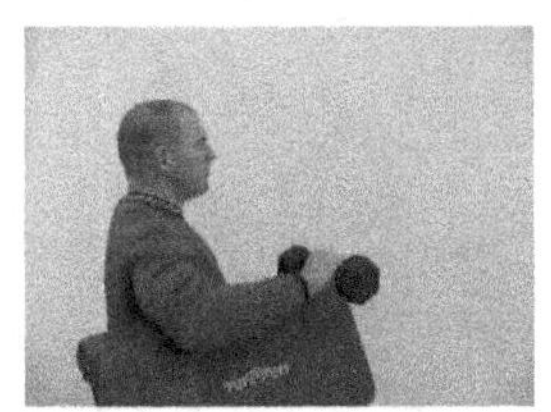 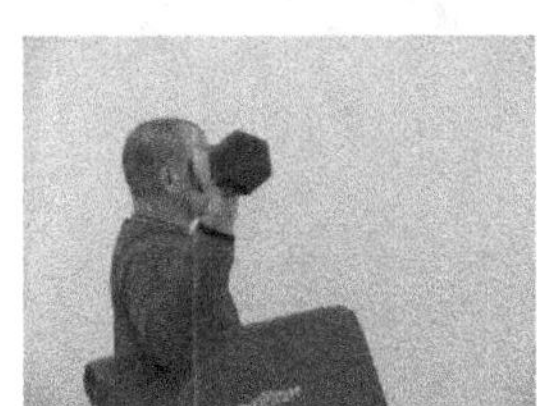

Sitting "L" Flys
2 X 12

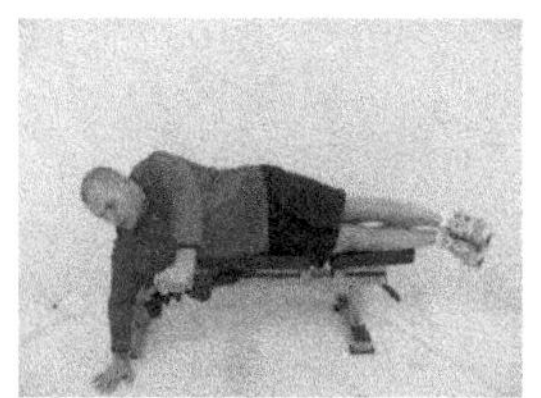 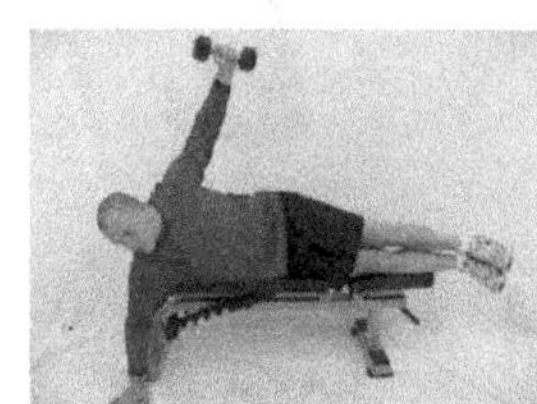

Lying Flys
2 X 12

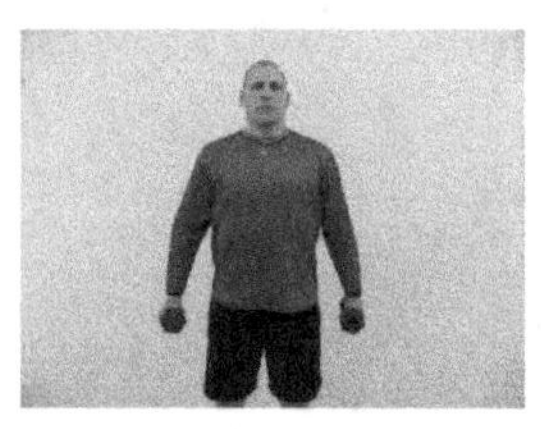 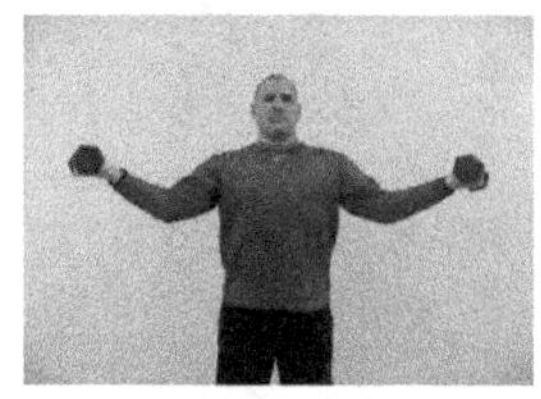

Quarter Eagles
2 X 12

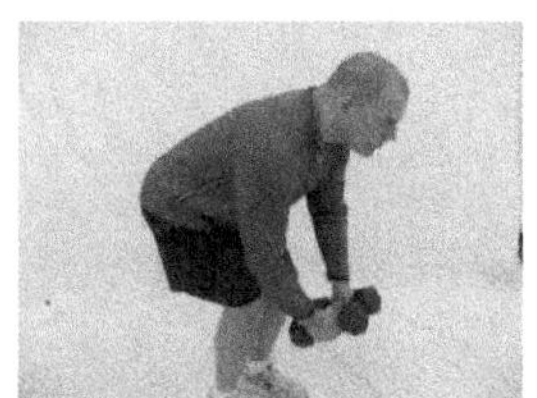 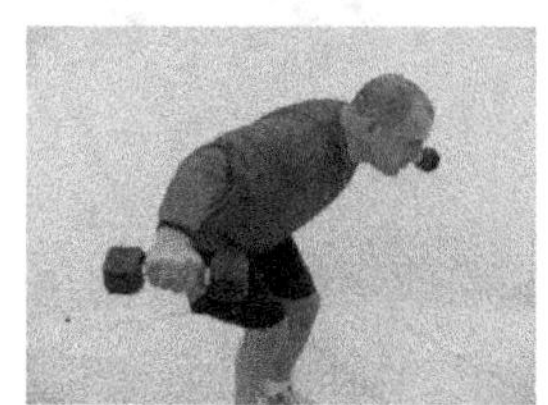

Rear Delt Raises
2 X 12

Bio

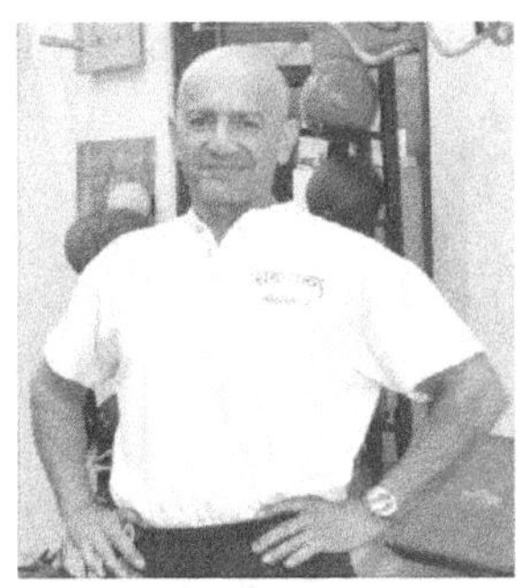

Coach Ahmad Soltani is a professional fitness trainer and the head coach at Hard Corps Athletics Inc., a fitness training/coaching facility located in Northern California. Since 1992 Coach Ahmad has been working as a fitness trainer and a fitness coach in a variety of disciplines including weight training, elastic band and tube training, calisthenics, TRX, SPIN, battle rope, boxing, archery and firearms. This book is the result of over 12 years of fitness training Wildland firefighters in Northern California and dealing with issues pledging law enforcement and first responders. Coach Ahmad routinely trains with local firefighters, police departments, SWAT teams and security personnel to get a first-hand look at the physical challenges, risks and demands they confront while performing their jobs.